I0695758

Table of Contents

Hypoglycemia is a condition caused by low blood glucose (blood sugar) levels. Glucose is the main way your body gets energy. The condition is most common in people with diabetes who have issues with medicine, food, or exercise. But sometimes people who don't have diabetes can also get low blood glucose. There are two kind of nondiabetic hypoglycemia:

Reactive hypoglycemia, which happens a few hours after you eat a meal

Fasting hypoglycemia, which might be linked to medicine or a disease

BREAKFAST

1. Biscuit Bake

Prep Time: 10 Minutes

Cook Time: 25 Minutes

Servings: 8

Ingredients

- 1 8 pk. store-bought biscuit dough (no flakey layers)
- 1 stick butter, melted
- 8 whole eggs, whisked
- 1/2 cup green onion, sliced thin
- 12 slices of bacon, cooked and cut in half
- 8 slices American cheese, unwrapped
- Optional honey or sriracha for drizzling

Intructions:

1. Preheat oven to 350° F.

2. Bake biscuits in 9 x 13 casserole dish until golden. Let cool for 2 - 3 minutes and remove the tops from all biscuits.

3. In a small saute pan, cook eggs over medium low heat. Season with salt and pepper. Make nice large curds in the egg using a rubber spatula and gently pushing the egg from the outside in. Slowly break up the eggs and remove from heat.

4. Start layering the sandwichess with scrambled eggs, topped with 3 - 4 pieces of bacon, and finished with American cheese.

5. Drizzle the inside of the biscuit tops with optional drizzle of honey or sriracha, then top biscuits. Brush tops of biscuits with remaining butter, cover with foil and bake for 8 - 10 minutes, until the cheese is melted.

6. Serve!

Prep Time: 10 Minutes

Cook Time: 1Hrs 5 Minutes

Servings: 6

Ingredients

- 6 English muffins
- 12 slices Canadian bacon
- 1 cup milk
- 4 eggs
- 1/2 teaspoon paprika
- 1/2 teaspoon onion powder
- 1 teaspoon garlic powder
- 1 teaspoon Kosher salt
- 1/2 teaspoon freshly ground black pepper
- Fresh chives, snipped, optional

For The Hollandaise Sauce:

- 3 egg yolks
- 1 tablespoon lemon juice
- 10 tablespoons unsalted butter, melted, but still warm
- 1/2 teaspoon Kosher salt

Instructions

1. Preheat oven to 350°F.

2. Separate English muffins and line them up vertically in a baking dish. Tuck slices of Canadian bacon in between the muffin halves.

3. In a medium bowl, whisk together eggs, milk, paprika, onion powder, garlic powder, and salt.

4. Pour evenly over muffins in baking dish. Cover dish tightly with foil and bake 30 minutes. Uncover and bake 30 minutes more.

5. During the last few minutes of baking, prepare the Hollandaise sauce:

6. Add egg yolks, lemon juice, and salt to a blender and blend at medium-high speed until lightened in color, about 30 seconds.

7. Lower blender speed and slowly drizzle in melted butter. Continue blending until all butter is incorporated.

8. Adjust lemon juice and salt as needed, drizzle over casserole, and enjoy! Sprinkle with fresh chives before serving, if desired.

Prep Time: 15 Minutes

Cook Time: 15 Minutes

Servings: 6

Ingredients8

- 1 chorizo, finely chopped
- 3 oz shredded cheese
- 1 tablespoon dried chives
- 1 teaspoon sweet paprika
- 1 teaspoon cumin
- Spray cooking oil
- Kosher salt and black pepper, to taste

For The Spicy Guac:

- 1 large avocado, mashed
- 1-2 teaspoons Kosher salt
- 1 teaspoon cayenne pepper
- 1 teaspoon garlic powder
- 1 tablespoon lemon juice
- Hot sauce to taste

Instructions

1. Finely chop chorizo. Add to a frying pan and cook on med-high heat for 3-4 minutes, then remove and set aside.
2. Switch fry pan to a lower heat. Add eggs and chives, muddling quickly until scrambled. Remove from pan and place in a bowl.
3. Preheat corn tortillas for 20-30 seconds in the microwave to help avoid splitting
4. Mix spices together thoroughly, then build the layers of the taquito: cheese, spices, chorizo, eggs, spices, and cheese.
5. Roll up each taquito and lay in air fryer tray with the seam down.
6. Spray with oil and cook for 6-8 minutes at 350°F, or until golden brown and crispy.
7. While taquitos are cooking, combine guac ingredients in a bowl and mash roughly with a fork.
8. Remove taquitos from air fryer and serve immediately, adding a generous amount of spicy guac, sour cream, and hot sauce to taste.

Prep Time: 10 Minutes

Cook Time: 45 Minutes

Servings: 6

Ingredients:

- 4 croissants, roughly chopped
- 1 cup orange marmalade
- 1 (8 oz) package cream cheese, at room temperature
- 1/2 cup granulated sugar
- 2 large eggs
- 1 cup whole milk
- Zest from one orange
- 1/2 teaspoon almond extract

Instructions

1. Preheat oven to 350°F and grease a 2 qt baking dish (8-inch square works well) with butter or nonstick spray.
2. In a large bowl, beat the cream cheese with an electric mixer until smooth and fluffy, about 3 minutes.

3. Add sugar and beat until fully incorporated, then add eggs, milk, orange zest, and almond extract and again mix to combine.

4. Place chopped croissants in prepared baking dish and place dollops of marmalade among them, stirring a bit to distribute if needed.

5. Pour cream cheese mixture over croissants, then cover dish tightly with foil.

6. Bake 30 minutes, then uncover and bake until top is golden brown and toothpick inserted in the center comes out clean, about 15 more minutes.

7. Let cool slightly before serving. Dust with powdered sugar, if desired, and serve. Enjoy!

Prep Time: 15 Minutes

Cook Time: 35 Minutes

Servings: 8

Ingredients:

- 1 small white or yellow onion
- 1 Tbsp butter
- 2 lb crumbled breakfast sausage of your choice
- 1 30-oz bag frozen shredded hash browns
- salt and pepper to taste
- 1/4 tsp garlic powder
- 1/4 tsp onion powder
- 2 cups shredded cheddar cheese
- 8 eggs
- 2 cups milk

Instructions

1. Add butter to large skillet and cook onions over medium heat for 3-5 minutes, adding salt and pepper to taste. Remove from pan and wipe it clean.

2. Add sausage to skillet and cook on medium high until brown, about 8 minutes. Remove from pan and add in potatoes. Reduce heat back to medium and cook for 5 minutes or so, flipping halfway. Add salt and pepper to taste.

3. In a large bowl whisk together eggs and milk. Add in more salt and pepper, as well as garlic powder and onion powder and whisk again to combine.

4. Grease a 9"x13" pan. Place hash browns on the bottom, followed by the onions, eggs, and sausage. Top with cheese and place in fridge for up to overnight if making ahead. If not bake uncovered for 30-35 minutes at 350°F until cheese is melted.

Prep Time: 10 Minutes

Cook Time: 20 Minutes

Servings: 6

Ingredients:

- 2 Tablespoons light olive oil, divided
- 2/3 cup diced yellow onion or 1 small yellow onion
- 2/3 cup diced celery or 2-3 celery ribs
- 1/2 cup diced carrot or 1 large carrot
- 1 teaspoon minced garlic or 2 medium garlic cloves
- 1/2 cup DeLallo Gluten-Free Corn & Rice Orzo
- 1–1/2 cups long-grain white rice
- 1 cup fresh cranberries
- 3 cups broth (chicken or vegetable)
- 3 sprigs fresh thyme or 1 tsp dried thyme
- Kosher Salt

Mix-ins:

- 1/3 cup slivered almonds, toasted
- 1 small Granny Smith apple, chopped
- 3 Tablespoons minced fresh curly parsley

- 1/4 c pomegranate arils, optional
- 1 Tablespoon lemon juice
- Kosher salt to taste
- Ground black pepper to taste

Instructions

1. Heat a 4-quart Instant Pot using the SAUTE mode. Add 1 Tablespoon olive oil and swirl to coat the bottom. Saute the onion, celery, and carrot for several minutes, stirring occasionally until vegetables are tender.
2. Add garlic, orzo, and white rice to Instant Pot and saute an additional 2-3 minutes until rice is slightly toasted. Turn saute off and add cranberries, broth, and thyme and a pinch of salt.
3. Lock the Instant Pot lid and set the vent to closed. Select MANUAL mode and cook rice on high pressure for 3 minutes then allow a natural release for 10-12 minutes.
4. Unlock the Instant Pot lid and discard thyme sprigs. Fluff pilaf with a fork and toss in the toasted almonds, apple, parsley, and pomegranate arils (optional). Sprinkle with lemon juice and season with salt and pepper, to taste.

5. Store in an airtight container in the fridge for 3-4 days.

6. Heat a medium-sized saucepan (or Dutch oven) over high heat. Add 1 Tablespoon olive oil and swirl to coat the bottom. Saute the onion, celery, and carrot for several minutes, stirring occasionally until vegetables are tender.

7. Add garlic, orzo, and white rice to the pan and saute an additional 2-3 minutes until rice is slightly toasted. Turn off the heat and add cranberries, broth, thyme and a pinch of salt.

8. Bring to a boil. Then turn down the heat, cover the saucepan with a lid, and simmer on low for 20-25 minutes or until liquid is absorbed.

9. Remove from heat and discard the thyme sprigs. Fluff pilaf with a fork and toss in the toasted almonds, apple, parsley, and pomegranate arils (optional). Sprinkle with lemon juice and season with salt and pepper, to taste.

Prep Time: 12 Minutes

Cook Time: 28 Minutes

Servings: 10

Ingredients:

- 1 3/4 cups (180-185g) gluten free oat flour
- 1/2 cup (55-56g) fine blanched almond flour
- 2 teaspoons baking soda
- 1 teaspoon baking powder
- 1/4 teaspoon kosher salt
- 1/2 teaspoon cinnamon
- 1/8 teaspoon nutmeg
- 2 Tablespoons coconut sugar or brown sugar, optional
- 1/2 cup non dairy milk at room temp or warm (so coconut oil doesn't solidify)
- 2 teaspoons lemon juice or apple cider vinegar
- 2 Tablespoons melted coconut oil or refined avocado oil
- 1/2 – 2/3 cup pure maple syrup or honey (adjust to desired sweetness)
- 1 cup fresh cranberries

- 1 Tablespoon orange zest

- 1 large egg or flax egg (see notes)

- 3 Tablespoons orange juice

- Optional Topping: orange slices

- Optional Batter Mix-ins – Chopped nuts or 1 Tablespoon ground flaxseed, 1/4 teaspoon orange extract for extra orange flavor.

Instructions

1. Preheat the oven to 350F. Line a 12-count muffin pan with liners or spray with cooking spray, set aside.

2. In a large mixing bowl, sift together the dry ingredients – oat flour, almond flour, baking soda, baking powder, salt and cinnamon, nutmeg and optional coconut sugar.

3. In a large measuring cup or medium-sized bowl, whisk together the non dairy milk, lemon juice, oil, and maple syrup. Set aside and let it sit for 10 minutes to create a "buttermilk" like wet batter.

4. Next, chop (by hand of food processor) the cranberries into small pieces. Transfer to a small bowl and mix with orange zest. Set aside.

5. Whisk the egg and orange juice into the wet mixture (buttermilk). Then, working in batches, gently combine wet ingredients into the dry ingredients. Do not over-mix.

6. Fold in the cranberry and orange zest mixture. Let the batter sit and thicken for 10 minutes. Pour batter into a greased or lined muffin pan filling ¾ full. Top batter with optional orange slices.

7. Bake at 350F for 18-22 minutes or until a toothpick inserted into the center comes out clean.

8. Remove muffins from the oven and let cool in muffin pan for 5 minutes before removing muffins to a cooling rack.

9. Store in an airtight container at room temperature for up to 2 days or in the fridge for up to 1 week.

Prep Time: 20 Minutes

Cook Time: 40 Minutes

Servings: 7

Ingredients:

- 3–4 cups of berries of choice – blueberries, raspberries, and/or blackberries.
- 1 cup (about 4 stalks) diced rhubarb
- 2 Tablespoons raw sugar or maple syrup
- 1/3–1/2 cup (around 70 grams) gluten free oat flour
- 1/4 cup coconut sugar or brown sugar
- 1 1/2 cups gluten free rolled oats
- 1 teaspoon cinnamon
- 1/4 teaspoon salt
- 6 Tablespoons solidified soy free vegan butter or refined coconut oil, diced

Instructions

1. Preheat the oven to 375° F.

2. Heat a large skillet on medium-low heat. Cook rhubarb with 2 teaspoons of sugar or maple syrup for 6-8 minutes or until it softens.

3. In a large bowl, combine the flour, sugar, oats, cinnamon, and salt. Add the butter (or solidified oil), and mix with two hands until a crumble texture is formed. Set aside.

4. Layer the rhubarb, berries, and crumble topping mixture into a cast iron pan or casserole dish.

5. Bake for 40-45 minutes or until bubbly. Note – If the edges start to burn before 40 minutes, cover with foil and continue to bake.

6. Store in an airtight container in the fridge for up to 5 days or freeze for up to 3 months.

7. To reheat, cover with foil and place in the oven at 350°F / 180°C until warmed through.

Prep Time: 35 Minutes

Cook Time: 55 Minutes

Servings: 9

Ingredients:

- 18–20 (250 grams) gluten free/vegan chocolate cookies (such as Glutino chocolate Vanilla Creme or dark chocolate cookies)
- 3–4 Tablespoons melted refined coconut oil or vegan butter (adjust as needed to allow the batter to hold together)

For the filling:

- 1 cup non dairy milk
- 3–4 Tablespoons fine cane sugar (adjust to desired sweetness)
- 1 1/2 Tablespoons cornstarch
- 1 1/2 teaspoons vanilla extract, divided

Pinch of salt:

- 1 can (13.5 ounces) coconut cream, chilled at least 6- 24 hours to thicken
- 2 (13.5 ounce) cans coconut milk, chilled at least 6- 24 hours to thicken
- 1/2 cup powdered sugar or fine cane sugar (powdered sugar will have a sweeter taste)
- Optional: 1/2 teaspoon butter extract for a "cream cheese" taste
- 21 (~12 ounces) gluten free chocolate vanilla creme cookies or dark chocolate cookies, crushed (See notes for vegan cookie brand recommendations)
- Optional: handful of dark chocolate chips

Instructions

To Prepare the Crust:

1. Place the cookies in the bowl of a food processor or blender. Pulse until a crumb-like texture is formed.
2. Add the melted oil/butter, and pulse again until well combined. If the batter is too dry, add an additional ½ to 1 Tablespoon of melted oil, and pule again.
3. Using hands or a measuring cup, press the crumb batter into the bottom of a pie pan and around the edges/sides.

4. Place the crust in the fridge for at least 30 minutes before filling.

To Prepare the filling:

1. Prepare the pudding. In a small saucepan, whisk the milk, sugar, cornstarch, 1 teaspoon of vanilla extract, and a pinch of salt on medium heat to combine. Simmer for 5-7 minutes, stirring frequently. Remove the saucepan from the heat, and let it cool in the fridge for 30-45 minutes or until the pudding has set.

2. While the pudding chills, prepare the coconut whipped cream filling. Place the solid cream portion of the coconut milk and cream in a stand mixer or mixing bowl. Discard the remaining liquid from the can. The cream should have a thick, cream cheese-like texture.

3. Add the powdered sugar, ½ teaspoon of vanilla extract, and optional butter extract to the cream. Whip/beat on medium speed for 2 minutes or until the batter is mixed thoroughly and light in texture. Place in the fridge.

4. Prepare the topping. Place the chocolate vanilla creme cookies in a bag or food processor, and pulverize until the cookies are crushed and crumbly. Set aside.

5. Remove the pudding and coconut cream mixture from the fridge. Fold the pudding mixture into the coconut

cream mixture, and stir until well combined. Adjust to desired sweetness.

6. Pour the pie filling batter into the chilled pie crust. Using the back of a spoon, spread the batter evenly, almost to the edge of the crust.

7. Top with the cookie crumbs and optional chocolate chips.

8. Freeze for 20 minutes to simplify cutting/serving, or place the pie in the refrigerator until ready to eat. Alternatively, freeze for 1+ hours for more of an ice cream cake/frozen pie texture. Freezing Tip – If using our homemade crust (recipe below) be sure to let it thaw out on the counter for 30 minutes before slicing.

9. Store in the fridge for 3-5 days or freezer for up to 3 months.

10. Nutrition below is for entire pie with cookie crust.

10. Chocolate Peanut Butter Cornflake Cookies

Prep Time: 10 Minutes

Cook Time: 20 Minutes

Servings: 18

Ingredients:

- 4 ounces dark chocolate
- 3/4 cup creamy peanut butter or nut/seed butter of choice
- 2/3 cup honey or agave nectar
- 1/2 teaspoon vanilla extract
- 3 cups plain cornflakes
- 1 cup unsweetened shredded coconut flakes + extra for topping
- Sea salt flakes to taste
- Optional: 3 Tablespoons chopped nuts

Instructions

1. Line a baking sheet with parchment paper. Set aside.

2. Heat a large saucepan over medium-high heat. Add the dark chocolate, nut butter, and honey, stirring to combine.

3. Heat the mixture until it comes to a boil. Remove the saucepan from the heat, and stir in the vanilla.

4. Working quickly, use a silicone spatula to gently stir in the remaining ingredients (cornflakes, shredded coconut, and optional chopped nuts) until they are well-coated with the chocolate mixture.

5. Using a large spoon or ice cream scoop, shape the batter into clusters, and place them on the baking sheet. Tip – be sure to use a smaller baking sheet so you can fit in the fridge or freezer later!

6. Sprinkle the cookies with extra coconut and sea salt flakes, if desired.

7. Place the cookies in the fridge to cool for 15-20 minutes before removing them from the baking sheet.

8. Best stored in the fridge for up to 1 week or freezer for up to 4 weeks.

11. Instant Pot Rice Pilaf with Orzo

Prep Time: 10 Minutes

Cook Time: 20 Minutes

Servings: 6

Ingredients:

- 2 Tablespoons light olive oil, divided
- 2/3 cup diced yellow onion or 1 small yellow onion
- 2/3 cup diced celery or 2-3 celery ribs
- 1/2 cup diced carrot or 1 large carrot
- 1 teaspoon minced garlic or 2 medium garlic cloves
- 1/2 cup DeLallo Gluten-Free Corn & Rice Orzo
- 1–1/2 cups long-grain white rice
- 1 cup fresh cranberries
- 3 cups broth (chicken or vegetable)
- 3 sprigs fresh thyme or 1 tsp dried thyme
- Kosher Salt

Mix-ins:

- 1/3 cup slivered almonds, toasted

- 1 small Granny Smith apple, chopped
- 3 Tablespoons minced fresh curly parsley
- 1/4 c pomegranate arils, optional
- 1 Tablespoon lemon juice
- Kosher salt to taste
- Ground black pepper to taste

Instructions

1. Heat a 4-quart Instant Pot using the SAUTE mode. Add 1 Tablespoon olive oil and swirl to coat the bottom. Saute the onion, celery, and carrot for several minutes, stirring occasionally until vegetables are tender.
2. Add garlic, orzo, and white rice to Instant Pot and saute an additional 2-3 minutes until rice is slightly toasted. Turn saute off and add cranberries, broth, thyme and a pinch of salt.
3. Lock the Instant Pot lid and set the vent to closed. Select MANUAL mode and cook rice on high pressure for 3 minutes then allow a natural release for 10-12 minutes.
4. Unlock the Instant Pot lid and discard thyme sprigs. Fluff pilaf with a fork and toss in the toasted almonds, apple, parsley, and pomegranate arils (optional).

Sprinkle with lemon juice and season with salt and pepper, to taste.

5. Store in an airtight container in the fridge for 3-4 days.

Stovetop Directions:

1. Heat a medium-sized saucepan (or Dutch oven) over high heat. Add 1 Tablespoon olive oil and swirl to coat the bottom. Saute the onion, celery, and carrot for several minutes, stirring occasionally until vegetables are tender.

2. Add garlic, orzo, and white rice to the pan and saute an additional 2-3 minutes until rice is slightly toasted. Turn off the heat and add cranberries, broth, thyme and a pinch of salt.

3. Bring to a boil. Then turn down the heat, cover the saucepan with a lid, and simmer on low for 20-25 minutes or until liquid is absorbed.

4. Remove from heat and discard the thyme sprigs. Fluff pilaf with a fork and toss in the toasted almonds, apple, parsley, and pomegranate arils (optional). Sprinkle with lemon juice and season with salt and pepper, to taste.

Prep Time: 8 Minutes

Cook Time: 30 Minutes

Servings: 6

Ingredients:

- 1 3/4 cups (180-185g) gluten free oat flour
- 1/2 cup (55-56g) fine blanched almond flour
- 2 teaspoons baking soda
- 1 teaspoon baking powder
- 1/4 teaspoon kosher salt
- 1/2 teaspoon cinnamon
- 1/8 teaspoon nutmeg
- 2 Tablespoons coconut sugar or brown sugar, optional
- 1/2 cup non dairy milk at room temp or warm (so coconut oil doesn't solidify)
- 2 teaspoons lemon juice or apple cider vinegar
- 2 Tablespoons melted coconut oil or refined avocado oil
- 1/2 – 2/3 cup pure maple syrup or honey (adjust to desired sweetness)
- 1 cup fresh cranberries

- 1 Tablespoon orange zest
- 1 large egg or flax egg (see notes)
- 3 Tablespoons orange juice
- Optional Topping: orange slices
- Optional Batter Mix-ins – Chopped nuts or 1 Tablespoon ground flaxseed, 1/4 teaspoon orange extract for extra orange flavor.

Instructions

1. Preheat the oven to 350F. Line a 12-count muffin pan with liners or spray with cooking spray, set aside.
2. In a large mixing bowl, sift together the dry ingredients – oat flour, almond flour, baking soda, baking powder, salt and cinnamon, nutmeg and optional coconut sugar.
3. In a large measuring cup or medium-sized bowl, whisk together the non dairy milk, lemon juice, oil, and maple syrup. Set aside and let it sit for 10 minutes to create a "buttermilk" like wet batter.
4. Next, chop (by hand of food processor) the cranberries into small pieces. Transfer to a small bowl and mix with orange zest. Set aside.

5. Whisk the egg and orange juice into the wet mixture (buttermilk). Then, working in batches, gently combine wet ingredients into the dry ingredients. Do not over-mix.

6. Fold in the cranberry and orange zest mixture. Let the batter sit and thicken for 10 minutes. Pour batter into a greased or lined muffin pan filling ¾ full. Top batter with optional orange slices.

7. Bake at 350F for 18-22 minutes or until a toothpick inserted into the center comes out clean.

8. Remove muffins from the oven and let cool in muffin pan for 5 minutes before removing muffins to a cooling rack.

9. Store in an airtight container at room temperature for up to 2 days or in the fridge for up to 1 week.

Prep Time: 20 Minutes

Cook Time: 40 Minutes

Servings: 5

Ingredients:

- 4 Tablespoons refined avocado oil or olive oil
- 1 1/2 cups chopped onions
- 1 pound (~3-4 cups) Cremini or white button mushrooms, sliced
- Optional: 1/3 cup dry white wine
- 2 teaspoons dried dill weed or 1 1/2 Tablespoons fresh dill, finely chopped
- 1 Tablespoon hot paprika
- Optional: Pinch of smoked paprika
- 1 Tablespoon tamari sauce or coconut aminos
- 2 1/2 cups vegetable or chicken broth
- 1 cup non-dairy milk
- 3 Tablespoons arrowroot flour (See notes)
- 1 teaspoon kosher salt
- Ground black pepper to taste
- 2 teaspoons lemon juice

- 1/4 cup chopped fresh parsley
- 1/2 cup full-fat coconut milk, canned and chilled

Instructions

1. Heat a large pot over medium heat. Place butter in a pot and melt, coating the pan.
2. Place the onions in the pot, and sauté for 5 minutes. Add the sliced mushrooms, and sauté for an additional 5 minutes until mushrooms are browned and coated in butter. Onions will brown as well.
3. Stir in the wine, dill, paprika, tamari sauce, and broth. Reduce heat to low, cover, and simmer for 15 minutes.
4. In a separate small bowl, whisk the non-dairy milk and arrowroot flour. Pour the flour and milk mixture into the soup, and stir thoroughly to blend. Cover pot, and simmer for 15 more minutes, stirring occasionally.
5. Finally, stir in the salt, ground black pepper, lemon juice, parsley, and solid coconut cream. Mix together, and allow to heat through over low heat, about 3 to 5 minutes. Do not boil.
6. Garnish with extra chopped parsley and cracked pepper. Serve immediately.
7. Store in an airtight container in the fridge for 3-4 days.

Prep Time: 10 Minutes

Cook Time: 15 Minutes

Servings: 5

Ingredients:

- 1 Tablespoon naturally refined avocado oil or pure olive oil
- 2/3 cup white onion, chopped
- 1 teaspoon minced garlic (about 2 small cloves)
- 1 1/2 cups frozen corn kernels, cooked or thawed
- 1 large bell pepper, chopped
- 3 to 3 1/2 cups cooked quinoa (see notes)
- 2 – 3 Tablespoons vegetable broth
- 1/4 teaspoon Kosher salt
- 1/4 teaspoon ground black pepper
- 1 teaspoon ground cumin
- 1/2 teaspoon chili powder (adjust to taste)
- 1 (10 ounce) can Original Diced Tomatoes & Green Chilies, drained (about 1 cup)* See notes for substitutes
- 1 1/2 cups shredded Mexican cheese or dairy free shredded cheese, divided

- Optional Garnishes: Fresh cilantro, chopped and fresh lime wedges for serving
- Optional Toppings: Diced avocado, sliced jalapeños, tortilla chips

Instructions

1. Heat a large oven-safe skillet on medium high heat. Add the oil to skillet and sauté onions until translucent, about 2 to 3 minutes. Stir in garlic and cook an additional 1 minute.
2. Add the corn and bell pepper to the pan and sauté for about 4 minutes, or until veggies are softened. Add the cooked quinoa, broth, salt, pepper, cumin, and chili powder (if using) and stir to combine.
3. Mix in drained canned tomatoes and green chiles. Reduce heat to medium low and cook for 5 minutes or until spices and sauces are absorbed with the quinoa and veggies. If the pan starts to dry out, add more broth.
4. Lastly, stir in 1 cup shredded cheese and continue to cook until melted, stirring occasionally.
5. (Optional) Preheat broiler to 450° F. Add the extra 1/2 cup cheese on top and place in the oven for 1 to 2

minutes or until the cheese is bubbly and edges are browned.

6. Remove from oven and let cool for 5 minutes before serving.

7. Top with cilantro and squeeze a fresh lime wedge to garnish. Serve with sliced jalapeños, avocado, and tortilla chips, if desired.

8. Store in the fridge for up to 4 days.

Prep Time: 5 Minutes

Cook Time: 15 Minutes

Servings: 2

Ingredients:

- 2 cucumber (peeled if desired)
- 6.50z wild caught lumb crab meat (fresh or canned)
- 2 tbsp chopped cilantro
- 1 tsp dried red pepper (flakes)
- 1/2 tsp minced garlic
- 2 –3 tsp sesame oil (divided)
- 2 tsp rice vinegar (more dressing if desired)
- splash of lime
- 1/2 to 1 whole avocado (sliced or chopped)
- 1 large plum
- sesame seeds (optional)
- sea salt / black pepper to taste

Instructions

1. Wash and dry your veggies/fruit. Next spiralize your cucumber or slice julienne style. Peel first if desired. Pat dry your cucumber spirals so they are oversaturated with water. Add spiralized cucumber to a bowl then mix in 1 tsp or more of sesame oil and rice vinegar.

2. In another small bowl, combine your crab meat, cilantro, pepper, garlic, vinegar, and 1 tsp sesame oil. Mix and add some fresh ground pepper if desired.

3. Slice up your plum and avocado.

4. Arrange all your ingredients in a large salad bowl or two small salad bowls. Season with salt/pepper and splash of lime. Garnish with sesame seeds.

Prep Time: 10 Minutes

Cook Time: 20 Minutes

Servings: 22

Ingredients:

- 3/4 cup gluten free rolled oats
- 1/3 cup dark chocolate chips
- 1/2 cup shredded unsweetened coconut
- 1 Tablespoon coconut sugar or brown sugar
- 1/3 cup chopped nuts

Pinch of cinnamon:

- 1/3 cup no stir creamy nut butter
- 1/3 cup honey or maple syrup
- Gluten free oat flour or plant based protein powder as needed (1-3 Tablespoons)

Instructions

1. In a large bowl, mix together the rolled oats, chocolate chips, coconut, coconut sugar, nuts, and a pinch of

cinnamon. Add the creamy nut butter and honey or maple syrup, and stir again to combine.

2. Adjust the amount of honey or maple syrup needed for the batter to stick together.

3. If batter is sticky, add 1-3 Tablespoons of gluten free oat flour or plant based protein powder, and mix together.

4. Place batter in the fridge for 20 minutes. This allows for easier rolling later.

5. Line a cookie sheet or large container with parchment paper. Set aside.

6. Remove the batter from the fridge, and roll into 1-1.5 inch balls. Place balls on a cookie tray. Then, freeze for 20-30 minutes.

7. Once chilled, transfer into a Ziploc bag.

8. Store in the fridge or freezer for up to 6 weeks.

Prep Time: 5 Minutes

Cook Time: 15 Minutes

Servings: 4

Ingredients:

For the Salmon:

- 10 −12 ounces fresh salmon (about 2 cups cooked flaked salmon) or two 5-ounce cans wild caught boneless salmon
- Olive oil to drizzle
- Kosher salt and pepper to taste

For the Dressing:

- 1/2 cup 2% plain yogurt / greek yogurt
- 2 teaspoons lemon juice
- 2 teaspoons raw honey
- 1 teaspoon Dijon mustard
- Kosher salt and black pepper to taste

For the Salad:

- 1 cup sliced strawberries

- 1 cup cucumber and/or celery, diced
- 1/2 large avocado (80 grams), diced
- 2 Tablespoons fresh parsley or basil, chopped
- Optional arugula for serving
- Optional Seasonings: cracked pepper, sea salt, lemon juice

Instructions

1. Preheat the oven to 400° F. Line a baking dish with parchment paper.
2. Use paper towels to pat the salmon dry. Drizzle with the olive oil, and generously season with salt and pepper. Bake for 10 -14 minutes, or 10 minutes per inch of salmon thickness. Use an instant-read thermometer to check that is has reached an internal temperature of 145° F. NOTE -> Thicker salmon will take closer to 14 minutes.
3. Remove from the oven, and let salmon rest for 5 minutes (It will continue to cook at rest). Then, flake it with a fork, and discard any skin. Place in a large mixing/serving bowl, and set aside. If using canned salmon, drain then flake with a fork, and place in a large bowl.

4. Prepare the dressing: In a small bowl, mix together the yogurt, lemon juice, honey, mustard, and salt, and pepper (to taste) until combined. Set aside.

5. Place strawberries, cucumber, and avocado in the bowl with the flaked salmon. Gently mix together. Add the yogurt dressing and fresh herbs and toss to combine. Taste and season as desired.

6. Serve on a bed of arugula, with gluten free crackers, with cooked quinoa, or as desired. See notes for lunch meal prep options.

Prep Time: 5 Minutes

Cook Time: 10 Minutes

Servings: 4

Ingredients:

For the Salad:

- 1/2 cup pecan halves (to be toasted)
- 5–6 cups (6 ounce bag) spinach leaves
- 2 cups (8 ounces) strawberries, sliced
- 1/2 cup (4 ounces) zucchini, sliced or julienne cut
- 1/2 large or 1 small avocado, diced
- 1/2 cup feta, crumbled
- Optional: 1/2 small red onion, sliced

For the Dressing:

- 1/3 cup olive oil or avocado oil
- 3 Tablespoons balsamic vinegar
- 1 Tablespoon honey
- 1 1/2 teaspoons dijon mustard
- 1 garlic clove (1/2 teaspoon), minced
- 1/4 teaspoon each sea salt and pepper

* Optional: 1 Tablespoon cherry juice (from jar or fresh)

Instructions

For the Pecans:

1. Preheat the oven to 350° F.
2. Spread the pecans on a baking sheet and toast/bake for 5 minutes or until they are golden and fragrant. Check oven halfway to ensure that the pecans do not burn. Remove from the oven and set aside.

For the Dressing:

1. In a small bowl (or covered jar), whisk together the dressing ingredients (oil, balsamic vinegar, honey, dijon mustard, garlic, salt and pepper and optional cherry juice) until well combined.
2. Prepare the Salad:
3. n a large serving bowl add the spinach, strawberries, zucchini, avocado, feta, toasted pecans, and optional red onion (see notes).
4. Drizzle the dressing on top, and toss lightly to combine.
5. Serve immediately. Refrigerate leftover salad dressing in an airtight container for up to 4-5 days. Always shake the dressing before serving.

Prep Time: 5 Minutes

Cook Time: 20 Minutes

Servings: 3

Ingredients:

Croutons:

- 1 to 1 1/2 cups diced gluten free bread (about 1 1/2 to 2 pieces)
- Olive oil to coat
- 1/2 teaspoon garlic powder
- Pinch of salt

For the Dressing:

- 1 large garlic clove (1–2 teaspoons minced garlic)
- 1 egg yolk (replace with 1 Tablespoon mayo or plain hummus for egg free option)
- 2 Tablespoons lemon juice
- 1 Tablespoon dijon mustard
- 1–2 teaspoons gluten free Worcestershire sauce (We us this one for gluten free option)
- 1/3 cup olive oil

- 1/4 – 1/3 cup freshly grated (fresh is key) Parmesan
- 1/4 teaspoon sea salt or kosher salt
- Black pepper to taste
- Spicy option! Add a pinch or two of cayenne or paprika

For Spicy Shrimp:

- 6–8 ounces medium shrimp, peeled, deveined
- 1/4 to 1/2 teaspoon chili powder
- 1/8 teaspoon onion powder
- 1/2 teaspoon pure olive oil or melted butter
- Pinch of sea salt or kosher salt
- Dash of ground pepper

For the Salad:

- 6 cups fresh torn romaine and spinach (leaves), combined
- Optional sliced vegetables – 1/2 cup cucumber or carrot
- Gluten Free Croutons (above)
- Spicy Baked Shrimp (above)
- 1/2 small avocado, sliced
- Shaved Parmesan to garnish

Instructions

How to Make the Gluten Free Croutons:

1. Preheat the oven to 350°F. Place the cubed bread in a mixing bowl. Drizzle the oil on top, and season with garlic powder and sea salt.
2. Toss the bread crumbs until coated. Then, place them on a baking sheet. Sprinkle optional grated Parmesan cheese on top.
3. Toast the bread in the oven for 8-10 minutes or until golden and crispy. While the croutons are baking, prep the dressing.

For the Dressing:

1. Press the garlic, and finely chop it into minced pieces.
2. In a small bowl, combine the egg yolk (or mayo/hummus), lemon juice, dijon, Worcestershire sauce, and garlic. Slowly drizzle in the extra virgin olive oil, whisking constantly.
3. Finish by whisking in freshly grated Parmesan cheese, salt, and pepper. Set aside while to prepare the shrimp, and remove the croutons from the oven to cool.

For the Spicy Shrimp:

1. Adjust the oven temperature to 450° F.

2. Toss the clean/peeled shrimp in olive oil and spices. Spread the shrimp on a medium baking sheet.

3. Bake the shrimp for 8-10 minutes, flipping once, halfway through cooking. The shrimp are done when the tails are browned and opaque throughout. Remove from the oven.

To Make Shrimp Caesar Salad:

1. Rinse and dry the torn romaine/spinach. Place it in a large serving bowl. Add additional sliced vegetables if desired, and toss to combine.

2. Add the cooled croutons, shrimp, avocado, and Parmesan shavings. Drizzle with Caesar dressing, and gently toss to combine.

3. Store covered in the fridge for up to 3 days.

Prep Time: 5 Minutes

Cook Time: 10 Minutes

Servings: 5

Ingredients

For the Avocado Egg Salad:

- 6 hard-boiled eggs
- 1/2 large avocado, diced (equivalent to 1/2 cup)
- 1 small bunch cilantro, chopped
- 3 ounces fire-roasted green chilies (canned, drained)
- 2 garlic cloves (1 teaspoon minced)
- 1/4 teaspoon paprika
- 1/2 teaspoon cumin
- dash of lime
- 1/3 cup red or green onion, chopped
- Salt to taste
- Black pepper to taste

For the Lettuce Wraps:

- 5 large lettuce leaves (ex: Romaine, butter lettuce, kale, or collard greens)

- Egg salad (above)
- 1 bell pepper, diced
- 1–2 jalapeños
- Salt to taste
- Fresh black pepper to taste
- 1 Fresh lime and juice
- Optional garnishes: chopped cilantro and/or spicy sprouts

Instructions

1. Slice the hard-boiled eggs in half. Remove the yolk, and place it in a food processor or blender. Keep the egg whites for later.
2. Combine the avocado, cilantro, green chilies, garlic, spices, a dash of lime juice, onion, salt, and pepper to taste in the food processor. Pulse/blend until a creamy, slightly chunky texture is formed. *See notes. Chop up a few of the extra egg whites from the hard-boiled eggs, and fold them into the egg salad mixture.
3. Clean the lettuce wraps, and place them on a towel. Pat dry. (See notes if using collard or kale leaves.)
4. Scoop ¼-⅓ cup of the avocado egg salad into each wrap.

5. Top with bell pepper slices, a dash of lime juice, red pepper flakes, jalapeño slices, salt, and pepper to taste. Garnish with optional spicy sprouts and/or chopped cilantro.

6. Storage – Keep the egg salad separate from the lettuce wraps in a sealed container in the fridge for up to 5 days.

21. Cinnamon Vanilla Protein Bites

Prep Time: 5 Minutes

Cook Time: 10 Minutes

Servings: 18

Ingredients:

- 3/4 cup of gluten free rolled oats or gluten free cereal of choice
- 1/4 cup (around 65–75 grams) Vanilla Protein Powder
- 1/2 cup almond flour or more oat flour if can't have nuts. (You can also just finely grind raw almonds) ·
- 1 heaping tablespoon ground Cinnamon (extra for coating)
- 1/4 to 1/3 cup nut butter or sunflower seed butter (creamy no stir works best)
- 1/2 tsp to 1 tsp Vanilla extract
- 1/4 to 1/3 cup maple syrup or honey if you are not vegan.

Instructions

1. Grind up your oats or cereal in a food processor and transfer into a mixing bowl. This is optional. You can keep them whole as well and adjust the addition of honey.
2. Add your almond meal, protein powder, cinnamon, and nut butter. Stir ingredients all together.
3. Alternatively (you can blend all at once by placing ingredients (minus the honey) in the food processor or blender and blend until a mealy batter is formed. Scrap sides and transfer to bowl (see blog post pictures).
4. Add in your honey and vanilla then mix again well with hands.
5. You might need to add more honey or nut butter if the batter gets to dry. (see notes)
6. Roll into 1-1.5 inch balls and place on a cookie tray or plastic ware with parchment paper underneath.
7. Let them freeze for 20-30 minutes then transfer into a Ziploc bag.
8. Dust with additional cinnamon and vanilla protein if desired.
9. Keep in fridge or freezer for up to 6 weeks.

Prep Time: 15 Minutes

Cook Time: 40 Minutes

Servings: 4

Ingredients:

- 5–6 cups of cauliflower florets (or 3–4 cups cauliflower rice). See notes.
- 2– 3 tbsp curry powder or curry seasoning (turmeric is usually included in curry seasoning/powder)
- 1 tsp garlic powder
- 1/2 tsp cumin
- 1/2 tsp paprika
- 1/4 tsp sea salt
- 2–3 tbsp olive oil
- 3/4 cup chopped red onion
- 1 tsp minced garlic
- 2 tsp olive oil or avocado oil
- 8 kale leaves, chopped
- 2 cups chopped carrots
- 4 cups vegetable broth

- 1 cup almond milk or coconut milk (the drinking kind works best and is smoother).
- 1/2 tsp red pepper or chili flakes (use less for a milder flavor)
- 1/2 tsp black pepper

Instructions

1. Preheat oven to 400F.
2. In a small bowl, toss cauliflower florets with curry powder, garlic powder, cumin, paprika, salt, and 3 tbsp oil.
3. Spread the cauliflower florets on a baking dish or roasting pan. Place in oven and roast for 20 -22 minutes, until tender but slightly under cooked. Remove and set aside to cool.
4. While the cauliflower is cooling, chop the remaining vegetables on a cutting board.
5. Next, place cauliflower florets in a Food Processor or blender and pulse a few times until the cauliflower resembles grains of rice. See picture in post.
6. Once all the cauliflower is riced and kale/veggies are chopped, prepare your cooking pot.

7. Place onion, 2 tsp oil, and minced garlic in large stock pot. Saute for 5 minutes until fragrant.

8. Next, add in broth, milk, veggies, cauliflower rice, red chili pepper and black pepper.

9. Bring to a boil, then immediately reduce heat to medium-low and simmer for another 20 minutes or so, until veggies are cooked.

10. Taste for seasoning and add dash of sea salt before serving, if desired.

Prep Time: 45 Minutes

Cook Time: 2hr 20 Minutes

Servings: 18

Ingredients:

- 2 large blood oranges or navel oranges, thinly sliced
- 1/4 cup coconut sugar or granulated sugar substitute
- 1/2 teaspoon ground cinnamon
- pinch of ground ginger
- dash of sea salt

Instructions

1. Preheat oven to 200°F.
2. Wash and dry oranges, then cut into very thin slices (as thin as possible). Lay them flat on a baking sheet with parchment paper.
3. In a small bowl, mix your spices and sugar.
4. Sprinkle evenly over orange slices.
5. Dry in the oven at 200°F. For 2 1/2 to 3 hours. If your orange slices are thick, they will take longer.

6. After removing them from the oven, add more spices
    and/or sugar, if desired.

7. Store in a cool dry place. Ziplock works great!

24. Paleo Cranberry Chicken

Prep Time: 25 Minutes

Cook Time: 45 Minutes

Servings: 5

Ingredients:

For the Marinade:

- 1/3 cup cranberries
- 2 tbsp olive oil
- 2 tbsp gluten free tamari sauce or coconut aminos (optional)
- 2 tbsp maple syrup
- 1/4 cup balsamic vinegar
- 1/4 tsp sea salt
- 1/4 tsp black peppers
- 2 garlic cloves (or 1 tsp minced)

For the Cranberry Chicken:

- lbs chicken thighs or breasts, with skin on (around 4 to 6 chicken thighs or breast) See notes for lower fat option

- 3–5 sprigs fresh thyme and extra to garnish (you may used a sprinkle of dried herbs to substitute)
- 1/3 cup to 1/2 cup fresh cranberries (or previously frozen)
- 1 tbsp each maple syrup and balsamic vinegar mixed together to coat chicken during roasting

Instructions

1. Prep – Clean your chicken, then place in a roasting or baking dish. Set aside.

Make the Balsamic Chicken Marinade:

2. Blend all the balsamic chicken marinade ingredients listed above in a food processor or blender until liquified and smooth.
3. Pour marinade over the chicken thighs, coating evenly.
4. Cover and place in fridge to marinate for 30 minutes or up to 24 hrs. (Overnight creates great flavor!)
5. Once marinated, preheat oven to 375 F.
6. Remove chicken from fridge.
7. Add extra 1/3 c to 1/2 cup cranberries, 2 – 3 sprigs of thyme or a sprinkle of dried Italian herbs to the dish. Spread it out evenly on and around the chicken.

8. Bake skin side down first for 25-35 minutes depending on the size of chicken thighs.

9. Remove and turn skin side up. Check for doneness. Then brush each chicken skin with the maple syrup/balsamic vinegar combo.

10. Add more seasoning (like dried herbs, salt, pepper) to the top if desired. NOTE: If using fresh herbs, wait to add until after you remove the chicken from the oven.

11. Depending on the thickness of your chicken thighs, either bake a little longer skin side up, then broil. Or if chicken is almost done and not pink, then skip extra baking and just broil for about 3-4 minutes or until skin is crispy and chicken is cooked evenly inside. Check to make sure the internal temperature of the thickest chicken thigh reaches 165F.

12. If using boneless chicken, cooking time will vary on thickness of chicken breast. Check around 35 minute's total.

13. After thoroughly cooked, remove from oven. Spoon the sauce from the pan onto each chicken thigh/breast and a pinch of black pepper or cracked pepper.

14. Serve with the roasted cranberries on top and any extra fresh herbs desired.

Prep Time: 25 Minutes

Cook Time: 1hr 35 Minutes

Servings: 5

Ingredients:

- 1 pound medium shrimp, peeled and deveined, tails removed (fresh or frozen then thawed) (see notes below for fresh shrimp)
- 1 Tablespoon olive oil (or avocado oil)
- 1 teaspoon minced garlic
- 1/2 cup chopped onion
- 1 bell pepper, chopped (about 1/2 to 2/3 cup)
- 14.5 ounce can fire roasted stewed tomatoes (diced work best)
- 1/2 cup chunky salsa
- kosher salt and black pepper to taste
- 1/2 teaspoon cumin
- 1/2 teaspoon chili powder or ancho chili powder
- 1/4 teaspoon paprika or cayenne pepper
- 2 Tablespoons chopped cilantro (extra for plating)

- Optional toppings – chopped green onion, sour cream, avocado, jalapeño pepper, etc.
- Tortillas to serve (gluten free corn tortillas or grain free low carb tortillas)

Instructions

1. First, prepare the shrimp if they are not already thawed. If using frozen shrimp, quickly thaw in water for 10 minutes before peeling. Pat the shrimp dry with paper towels.
2. Layer the shrimp at the bottom of the crockpot/slow cooker. Drizzle 1 tablespoon olive oil on top. Add the garlic, chopped onion and bell pepper, and toss to combine.
3. Add the drained canned fire roasted tomatoes, salsa, salt, pepper, cumin, chili powder, and paprika to the crockpot. Mix together until seasonings are well combined with shrimp and vegetables.
4. Place slow cooker (crock pot) on low for 2-3 hours or on high for 90 minutes to 2 hours. Stir once, about halfway through cooking.

5. Check on shrimp after about 1 hour of cooking on high. If they look almost done, place on medium for another 30 minutes to an hour.

6. Shrimp are done and cooked through once opaque, looking similar to that of steamed shrimp.

7. Serve with gluten free tortillas and fillings/toppings of choice. Ex: chopped green onions, avocado, jalapeño, and extra cilantro to garnish.

8. These tacos are best enjoyed right away.

Prep Time: 5 Minutes

Cook Time: 20 Minutes

Servings: 2

Ingredients:

Croutons:

- 1 to 1 1/2 cups diced gluten free bread (about 1 1/2 to 2 pieces)
- Olive oil to coat
- 1/2 teaspoon garlic powder
- Pinch of salt

For the Dressing:

- 1 large garlic clove (1–2 teaspoons minced garlic)
- 1 egg yolk (replace with 1 Tablespoon mayo or plain hummus for egg free option)
- 2 Tablespoons lemon juice
- 1 Tablespoon dijon mustard
- 1–2 teaspoons gluten free Worcestershire sauce (We us this one for gluten free option)
- 1/3 cup olive oil

- 1/4 – 1/3 cup freshly grated (fresh is key) Parmesan
- 1/4 teaspoon sea salt or kosher salt
- Black pepper to taste
- Spicy option! Add a pinch or two of cayenne or paprika

For Spicy Shrimp:

- 6–8 ounces medium shrimp, peeled, deveined
- 1/4 to 1/2 teaspoon chili powder
- 1/8 teaspoon onion powder
- 1/2 teaspoon pure olive oil or melted butter
- Pinch of sea salt or kosher salt
- Dash of ground pepper

For the Salad:

- 6 cups fresh torn romaine and spinach (leaves), combined
- Optional sliced vegetables – 1/2 cup cucumber or carrot
- Gluten Free Croutons (above)
- Spicy Baked Shrimp (above)
- 1/2 small avocado, sliced
- Shaved Parmesan to garnish

Instructions

1. How to Make the Gluten Free Croutons:
2. Preheat the oven to 350°F. Place the cubed bread in a mixing bowl. Drizzle the oil on top, and season with garlic powder and sea salt.
3. Toss the bread crumbs until coated. Then, place them on a baking sheet. Sprinkle optional grated Parmesan cheese on top.
4. Toast the bread in the oven for 8-10 minutes or until golden and crispy. While the croutons are baking, prep the dressing.

For the Dressing:

1. Press the garlic, and finely chop it into minced pieces.
2. In a small bowl, combine the egg yolk (or mayo/hummus), lemon juice, dijon, Worcestershire sauce, and garlic. Slowly drizzle in the extra virgin olive oil, whisking constantly.
3. Finish by whisking in freshly grated Parmesan cheese, salt, and pepper. Set aside while to prepare the shrimp, and remove the croutons from the oven to cool.

For the Spicy Shrimp:

1. Adjust the oven temperature to 450° F.

2. Toss the clean/peeled shrimp in olive oil and spices. Spread the shrimp on a medium baking sheet.

3. Bake the shrimp for 8-10 minutes, flipping once, halfway through cooking. The shrimp are done when the tails are browned and opaque throughout. Remove from the oven.

To Make Shrimp Caesar Salad:

1. Rinse and dry the torn romaine/spinach. Place it in a large serving bowl. Add additional sliced vegetables if desired, and toss to combine.

2. Add the cooled croutons, shrimp, avocado, and Parmesan shavings. Drizzle with Caesar dressing, and gently toss to combine.

3. Store covered in the fridge for up to 3 days.

Prep Time: 5 Minutes

Cook Time: 10 Minutes

Servings: 11

Ingredients:

- 1/3 cup cashews (raw or dry roasted)
- 3/4 cup unsweetened plain dairy-free milk + additional as needed
- 1/2 cup olive oil, avocado oil, or grapeseed oil
- 4 teaspoons lemon juice
- 2 teaspoons apple cider vinegar
- Optional 1 teaspoon maple syrup or honey
- 1 teaspoon sea salt
- 1/2 teaspoon ground mustard
- 1/2 teaspoon onion powder
- 1/4 – 1/2 teaspoon garlic powder
- 1/4 teaspoon black pepper
- 2 teaspoons dried parsley or 1/4 cup chopped fresh parsley

For the Platter:

- Vegetables of choice, sliced. (Ex: Carrots, celery, broccoli, grape tomatoes, etc.)
- Herbs and lemon slices to garnish
- Optional: gluten free or paleo-friendly crackers

Instructions

For the Ranch Dressing:

1. Put the cashews in a spice grinder or small food processor, and pulse until powdered, about 30 to 60 seconds.
2. Put the cashew powder, milk, oil, lemon juice, vinegar, honey or maple syrup, salt, mustard, onion powder, garlic powder, and pepper in the blender, and blend for 2 minutes. The ingredients should emulsify and thicken slightly. Stir in the parsley.
3. Pour the dressing into an airtight bottle or container, cover, and refrigerator for at least 30 minutes to thicken and let the flavors develop.
4. Store in the refrigerator for up to 1 week. Shake or whisk the dressing before each use. Makes 1 1/2 cups.

For the Snack Platter:

1. Place 1/2 cup to 2/3 cup of vegan ranch in a small bowl. Place the bowl on a large serving plate. Add the fresh vegetables and/or gluten free crackers around it.

2. Garnish with lemon slices and herbs. Add cracked pepper on top of ranch, if desired. (See notes for a nut free option.)

Prep Time: 3 Minutes

Cook Time: 10 Minutes

Servings: 3

Ingredients:

For the Dressing:

- 1 large garlic clove (1–2 teaspoons minced garlic)
- 1 egg yolk (replace with 1 Tablespoon real mayonnaise or plain hummus for egg free option)
- 2 Tablespoons lemon juice
- 1 Tablespoon dijon mustard
- 1–2 teaspoons gluten free Worcestershire sauce (We us this one for gluten free option)
- 1/3 cup olive oil
- 1/4 – 1/3 cup freshly grated Parmesan (fresh is key)
- 1/4 teaspoon sea salt or kosher salt
- Black pepper to taste

For the Salad:

- 1 pound tomatoes, sliced quartered, or halved (Heirloom and cherry tomatoes)

- Fresh lemon slices – to preserve tomatoes
- 1/2 cup fresh basil or to taste
- 2–3 Tablespoons (18–24 grams) toasted pine nuts
- Shaved Parmesan or nutritional yeast for serving
- Kosher salt and black pepper, to taste

Instructions

For the Caesar Dressing:

1. Press the garlic, and finely chop it into minced pieces.
2. In a small bowl, combine the egg yolk (or mayonnaise/hummus), lemon juice, dijon, Worcestershire sauce, and garlic. Slowly drizzle in the extra virgin olive oil, whisking constantly.
3. Finish by whisking in freshly grated Parmesan cheese, salt, and pepper. Set aside while preparing the tomatoes. (See notes for dairy free option)

For the Tomato Salad:

1. Rinse and drain the tomatoes.
2. Arrange the sliced tomatoes on a large plate.
3. Drizzle the dressing on top. Layer lemon wedges between the tomato slices. Add fresh herbs, pine nuts, and shaved Parmesan. Season generously.

4. Serve immediately.

5. Storage – For the best results, we recommend serving the prepared salad fresh. If needed, it can be kept in the fridge for a few hours before the tomatoes start to become soggy.

Prep Time: 10 Minutes

Cook Time: 27 Minutes

Servings: 4

Ingredients:

- 4 medium zucchini
- 2 Tablespoons olive oil, divided
- 1/3 cup diced onion
- 1 pound ground turkey
- 1 teaspoon sea salt, divided
- 1/4 teaspoon black pepper
- 10-ounce can diced tomatoes with green chilies, drained
- 1 cup enchilada sauce
- 1 cup Mexican cheese blend

Instructions

1. Preheat the oven to 400° F. Line a baking sheet with foil or parchment paper.

2. Slice the zucchini lengthwise. Use a spoon or melon baller to scoop out the seedy parts of the centers of the zucchini to make wells.

3. Place the zucchini on the baking sheet, cut side up. Drizzle with 1 Tablespoon of the olive oil and sprinkle 1/4 teaspoon salt lightly over all the zucchini.

4. Roast the zucchini in the oven for 15-20 minutes or until fork tender.

5. Meanwhile, heat another Tablespoon of olive oil in a large non-stick skillet over medium-high heat. Add the diced onions. Saute for 7-10 minutes or until they begin to brown.

6. Add the ground turkey. Season with pepper and the remaining 3/4 teaspoon salt. Cook for about 10 minutes, breaking apart with a spatula until browned.

7. Stir in the diced tomatoes with green chilies and enchilada sauce. Increase heat to bring to a gentle boil, then simmer for 5-7 minutes, until excess sauce absorbs into the meat.

8. When the zucchini are done, remove from the oven and leave the oven at 400° F.

9. Use paper towels to pat any moisture from the zucchini boats. Spoon the turkey mixture inside, then sprinkle with cheese.

10. Bake for about 5 minutes, until the cheese is melted.

11. Storage: Keep in the refrigerator for up to 5 days. Or, freeze for 3-6 months.

Prep Time: 30 Minutes

Cook Time: 1hr 35 Minutes

Servings: 6

Ingredients:

- 1 Tablespoon olive oil
- 1/2 onion, finely diced
- 1 Tablespoon minced fresh garlic
- 1 (8 ounce) package sliced fresh mushrooms
- 1/2 teaspoon salt
- Optional extra diced veggies: 1/2 cup zucchini or bell pepper
- 1 jar (24 ounces) tomato basil spaghetti sauce (Delallo)
- 1 cup water
- 1/4 cup chicken or vegetable broth
- 12 ounces dry DeLallo gluten free brown rice spaghetti noodles or dry gluten free corn and rice spaghetti noodles
- 1/2 cup grated Parmesan cheese or nutritional yeast
- 1 (24 ounces) jar DeLallo Tomato Puree
- Fresh parsley or basil to taste

- Red pepper flakes, to taste
- Optional: 1 pound meat of choice (Ex. sausage, ground beef or turkey, etc.)

Instructions

1. Heat oil in a large skillet over medium-high heat. Add onion and garlic, and sauté until fragrant, about 2-3 minutes. Add the sliced mushrooms and salt. Cook on medium until mushrooms sweat and soften, about 3 minutes, deglazing skillet if needed.
2. Stir in the optional diced vegetables.
3. Pour one jar of the spaghetti sauce and the water/broth into the bottom of a slow cooker. Break the spaghetti noodles in half, and place them on top of the sauce. TIP -> Make sure the noodles are layered in alternating directions. (See blog photo.)
4. Add the cooked vegetable mixture to the slow cooker, mix to combine. Sprinkle with Parmesan cheese or nutritional yeast, and pour second jar of tomato purée on top.
5. Cover and cook on HIGH for 1-2 hours or on LOW for up to 2 ½ hours, stirring periodically (if possible). (See notes) Toss all of the ingredients together, and serve.

6. Keep leftovers in the fridge for 3-5 days.